70 Effective Meal Recipes to Prevent and Solve Your Overweight Problems:

Burn Calories Fast by Using Proper Dieting and Smart Nutrition

By

Joe Correa CSN

COPYRIGHT

ACKNOWLEDGEMENTS

This book is dedicated to my friends and family that have had mild or serious illnesses so that you may find a solution and make the necessary changes in your life.

70 Effective Meal Recipes to Prevent and Solve Your Overweight Problems:

Burn Calories Fast by Using Proper Dieting and Smart Nutrition

By

Joe Correa CSN

CONTENTS

ABOUT THE AUTHOR

After years of Research, I honestly believe in the positive effects that proper nutrition can have over the body and mind. My knowledge and experience has helped me live healthier throughout the years and which I have shared with family and friends. The more you know about eating and drinking healthier, the sooner you will want to change your life and eating habits.

Nutrition is a key part in the process of being healthy and living longer so get started today. The first step is the most important and the most significant.

INTRODUCTION

70 Effective Meal Recipes to Prevent and Solve Your Overweight Problems: Burn Calories Fast by Using Proper Dieting and Smart Nutrition

By Joe Correa CSN

These recipes came as a result of my own battle with controlling my weight and there is nothing in this world that would make me happier than to see them help someone else. Enjoy food every single day and witness your body change!

Being overweight is a serious health problem that often leads to different chronic diseases especially diseases related to heart, blood vessels, and diabetes. Despite the undeniable fact that a healthy lifestyle is being promoted like never before, experts say that by 2025, more that 50% of the population in the USA will be obese. In my own experience, the hardest part can be creating a proper mental state, and keep yourself on the path of weight control.

Dealing with extra weight can be mentally and physically exhausting, especially because it takes a longer time to lose all that weight. Extreme diets are unnecessary, you just have to eat what your body needs not what it wants. This is where most people usually give up but the secret is in eating delicious and healthy food so that you don't have to eat tastless food.

One day I decided to try something new and started eating differently. Slowly, I reduced my portion sizes and tried to eat as healthy as possible without stressing about it. And it worked! My body started to change without the terrible yo-yo effect. I was thrilled with my new results. To be honest, the changes were happening fast but atleast they were changes. I felt stronger and healthier every day which motivated me to eat even healthier. For months researched and experimented with different recipes that would make my diet more and more enjoyable besides being healthy! I love to eat and I'm not ashamed of it. I have realized that a healthy meal can be ten times more delicious than some processed junk we often turn to after a long day at work. If you're struggling with an eating problem like I did, I'm more than happy to tell you that a solution does exist and it tastes great, believe it or not! You don't have to give up eating and the pleasure that food brings to our lives just to lose some weight! On the contrary, allow the food to become your ally in defeating the extra weight you want to get rid of once and for all!

70 EFFECTIVE MEAL RECIPES TO PREVENT AND SOLVE YOUR OVERWEIGHT PROBLEMS: BURN CALORIES FAST BY USING PROPER DIETING AND SMART NUTRITION

1.   Greek Salad

Ingredients:

2 large tomatoes, chopped

1 large cucumber, sliced

1 small onion, chopped

1 cup of Feta cheese, crumbled

¼ cup of green olives, pitted and halved

2 tbsp of extra-virgin olive oil

2 tbsp of balsamic vinegar

3 tbsp of lemon juice, freshly squeezed

½ tsp of salt

¼ tsp of black pepper, ground

½ tsp of dried oregano, ground

Preparation:

Combine olive oil, vinegar, lemon juice, salt, pepper, oregano, and olives in a mixing bowl. Stir well to mix and set aside to allow flavors to mingle.

In a large bowl, combine cheese, tomatoes, cucumber, and onions. Drizzle with previously made dressing and toss to coat. Refrigerate for 20 minutes before serving. Enjoy!

Nutrition information per serving: Kcal: 163, Protein: 5.6g, Carbs: 8.2g, Fats: 12.6g

2.   Avocado Berry Smoothie

Ingredients:

1 ripe avocado, pitted, peeled and chopped

½ cup of frozen raspberries

¼ cup of frozen blueberries

1 tbsp of lemon juice, freshly squeezed

1 tbsp of honey

1 ½ cup of water

Preparation:

Combine all ingredients in a food processor and blend until smooth. Transfer the mixture to a serving glasses and refrigerate for at least 1 hour before serving. Enjoy!

Nutrition information per serving: Kcal: 157, Protein: 1.3g, Carbs: 18.2g, Fats: 9.9g

3.   Strawberry Salad with Spinach

Ingredients:

1 cup of fresh strawberries, chopped

3 small kiwis, peeled and chopped

1 cup of fresh spinach, finely chopped

½ cup of almonds, roughly chopped

1 tbsp of raspberry vinegar

4 tbsp of vegetable oil

1 tbsp of honey

1 tbsp of lemon juice

Preparation:

Combine lemon juice, honey, oil, and vinegar in a small bowl. Stir to mix and set aside.

Meanwhile, place strawberries, kiwis, spinach, and almonds in a large bowl. Toss to combine and drizzle with dressing and give it a final stir. Serve immediately.

Nutrition information per serving: Kcal: 339, Protein: 4.9g, Carbs: 24.5g, Fats: 26.7g

4.   Beef Stew with Eggplants

Ingredients:

10 oz of beef neck, chopped into bite-sized pieces

1 large eggplant, sliced

2 cups of fire-roasted tomatoes

½ cup of fresh green peas

1 cup of beef broth

4 tbsp of olive oil

2 tbsp of tomato paste, sugar-free

1 tbsp of Cayenne pepper, ground

½ tsp of chili pepper, ground

½ tsp of salt

Preparation:

Grease the bottom of a deep, heavy-bottomed pot with olive oil. Toss all ingredients in it and add about 1-1 ½ cup of water.

Cook for 2 hours over medium-low heat, or until the meat is fork-tender.

Nutrition information per serving: Kcal: 195, Protein: 15.3g, Carbs: 9.6g, Fats: 11.1g

5.   Coconut Quinoa Breakfast

Ingredients:

1 cup of white quinoa, pre-cooked

1 cup of coconut milk, unsweetened

¼ cup of raisins

1 tbsp of honey, raw

1 tbsp of flaxseeds

Preparation:

Place the quinoa in a deep pot. Pour 2 cups of water and bring it to a boil. Reduce the heat to low and add coconut milk and flaxseeds. Stir well and cook for 15 minutes. Remove from the heat and set aside to cool completely.

Stir in the raisins, and honey. Serve immediately.

Nutrition information per serving: Kcal: 462, Protein: 10.6g, Carbs: 56.8g, Fats: 23.3g

6.   Green Pepper Chicken Wings

Ingredients:

1 lb of chicken breasts, chopped

2 large potatoes, peeled and finely chopped

5 large green bell peppers, finely chopped

2 small carrots, sliced

2 ½ cups of chicken broth

1 large tomato, roughly chopped

¼ cup of fresh parsley, finely chopped

3 tbsp of extra-virgin olive oil

1 tbsp of cayenne pepper

1 tsp of chili pepper, freshly ground

1 tsp of salt

Preparation:

Preheat the oil in a large saucepan over a medium-high temperature. Place all the vegetables in one layer and top with chicken wings. Add chicken broth, Cayenne pepper, salt, and fresh parsley. Bring it to a boil then reduce the heat to low. Cover with a lid and cook for 1 hour, stirring constantly.

Serve warm.

Nutrition information per serving: Kcal: 325, Protein: 11.5g, Carbs: 44.5g, Fats: 12.8g

7.   Easy Lobster Recipe

Ingredients:

1 medium-sized lobster, whole (about 2lbs)

¼ cup of extra-virgin olive oil

1 tbsp of Cayenne pepper, ground

½ tsp of sea salt

¼ tsp of black pepper, ground

Preparation:

Preheat the oven to 350°F.

With a sharp knife, cut top side of lobster shells lengthwise.

Combine the olive oil with sea salt, Cayenne pepper, and ground black pepper. Place the lobster on a baking sheet and pull apart shells. Season the meat with this mixture.

Cook for about 10 minutes, until lightly golden color. Serve warm.

Nutrition information per serving: Kcal: 111, Protein: 20.6g, Carbs: 0.4g, Fats: 6.5g

8.   Garlic Chicken Breast

Ingredients:

2 chicken breast halves, skinless and boneless

½ cup of extra-virgin olive oil

3 garlic cloves, crushed

½ cup of fresh parsley, chopped

1 tbsp of lime juice, freshly squeezed

½ tsp of salt

Preparation:

Combine the olive oil with crushed garlic cloves, finely chopped parsley, fresh lime juice and some salt (about ¼ tsp will be enough). Wash and pat dry the meat and cut into 1 inch thick slices.

With a kitchen brush, spread the olive oil mixture over the meat. Let it stand for about 15 minutes.

Preheat the grill pan over a medium-high temperature. Add about 2 tablespoons of marinade in the grill pan. Place the meat in it and grill on both sides, until lightly charred.

Remove from the pan and serve with some fresh vegetables of your choice.

Nutrition information per serving: Kcal: 146, Protein: 33.2g, Carbs: 0.6g, Fats: 6.9g

9.   Coconut Peanut Butter Smoothie

Ingredients:

1 cup of coconut milk, unsweetened

1 tbsp of peanut butter, unsweetened

1 tbsp of honey, raw

¼ tsp of sea salt

Preparation:

Combine all ingredients in a blender and process until nicely smooth. Transfer the mixture to a serving glasses and refrigerate for 30 minutes before using. Garnish with finely chopped mint or nuts if you like. However, this is optional.

Nutrition information per serving: Kcal: Protein: 33.2g, Carbs: 0.6g, Fats: 6.9g

10.   Greek Dolmades

Ingredients:

40 wine leaves, fresh or in jar

1 cup of brown rice

½ cup of olive oil

3 garlic cloves, crushed

¼ cup of lemon juice, freshly squeezed

2 tbsp fresh mint

½ tsp of salt

Preparation:

Wash the leaves thoroughly, one at a time. Place on a clean working surface. Grease the bottom of a deep pot with oil and make a layer with wine leaves. Set aside.

In a medium-sized bowl, combine rice with 3 tablespoons of olive oil, garlic, mint, salt, and pepper. Place one wine leaf at a time on a working surface and add one teaspoon of filling at the bottom end. Fold the leaf over the filling towards the center. Bring the two sides in towards the center and roll them up tightly. Gently transfer to a pot.

Add the remaining olive oil, 2 cups of water, and lemon juice. Cover and cook for 30 minutes, over medium-high heat.

Remove from the pot and chill overnight in the refrigerator.

Nutrition information per serving: Kcal: 313, Protein: 2.9g, Carbs: 30.4, Fats: 20.5g

11.　Mushroom Kebab

Ingredients:

1 lb of lean grass-fed veal cuts, chopped into bite-sized pieces

1 lb of chicken breast, boneless, skinless, and chopped into bite-sized pieces

12 oz button mushrooms, sliced

3 large carrots, sliced

2 tbsp of butter, softened

1 tbsp of olive oil

1 tbsp of Cayenne pepper

1 tsp of salt

½ tsp of black pepper, freshly ground

A bunch of fresh celery leaves, finely chopped

3 ½ oz celery root, finely chopped

Preparation:

Grease the bottom of a deep pot with olive oil. Add veal chops, sliced carrot, salt, pepper, cayenne pepper, and celery root. Give it a good stir, add 2 cups of water, and cover with a lid.

Cook for about 45 minutes, or until the meat is half-cooked.

Uncover and add chicken breast, butter, and one more cup of water. Continue to simmer for 45 more minutes, or until the meat is fully cooked and tender.

Finally, add mushrooms and celery. I personally don't like to overcook the mushrooms so about 5 more minutes will be more than enough.

Serve warm.

Nutrition information per serving: Kcal: 373, Protein: 37.6g, Carbs: 11.3g, Fats: 20.2g

12. Parmesan Salad

Ingredients:

1 cup of Parmesan cheese, shredded

2 cups of Iceberg lettuce, chopped

1 small cucumber, chopped

½ cup of cherry tomatoes, halved

1 large bell pepper, chopped

3 tbsp of extra-virgin olive oil

½ tsp of sea salt

2 tbsp of fresh parsley, finely chopped

¼ tsp of black pepper, ground

Preparation:

Combine oil, parsley, salt, and pepper in a mixing bowl. Stir well and set aside.

Meanwhile, combine lettuce, cucumber, and tomatoes in a large bowl. Top with parmesan and drizzle with previously made dressing. Toss well to coat and serve.

Nutrition information per serving: Kcal: 200, Protein: 9.2g, Carbs: 7.8g, Fats: 16.1g

13.   Eggplant Stew

Ingredients:

4 medium-sized eggplants, halved

3 large tomatoes, finely chopped

2 red bell peppers, finely chopped and seeds removed

¼ cup of tomato paste

1 small bunch of fresh parsley, finely chopped

3 ½ oz of toasted almonds, finely chopped

2 tbsp of salted capers, rinsed and drained

¼ cup of extra-virgin olive oil

1 tsp of sea salt

Preparation:

Grease the bottom of a deep pot with two tablespoons of extra virgin olive oil. Make the first layer with halved eggplants tucking the ends gently to fit in.

Now, make the second layer with finely chopped tomatoes and red bell peppers. Spread the tomato paste evenly over the vegetables, sprinkle with finely chopped almonds and salted capers. Add the remaining olive oil, salt and pepper. Pour about 1 ½ cups of water and cover with a lid. Cook for about 2 hours over a medium temperature.

Nutrition information per serving: Kcal: 259, Protein: 7.5g, Carbs: 30.1g, Fats: 15.1g

14.   Pistachio Oatmeal

Ingredients:

1 cup of oatmeal

1 cup of water

2 tbsp of pistachios, unsalted

1 tsp of honey, liquid

1 cup of Greek yogurt

Preparation:

In a medium pot, combine quinoa and water. Bring it to a boil then reduce the heat to low and cook for another 15 minutes. Remove from the heat and let it cool for a while. Add pistachios and honey and give it a good stir. Top with Greek yogurt and serve.

Nutrition information per serving: Kcal: 169, Protein: 10.1g, Carbs: 23.5g, Fats: 4.2g

15. Asian Asparagus Salad

Ingredients:

1 lb of wild asparagus, trimmed

1 cup of spring onions, chopped

1 cup of red cabbage, chopped

1 tbsp of white wine vinegar

1 tbsp of canola oil

½ tsp of ginger, freshly grated

1 tsp of chili pepper, ground

½ tsp of salt

¼ tsp of black pepper, ground

Preparation:

Place the asparagus in a pot of boiling water. Cook for about 3-5 minutes, or until soften. Remove from the heat and soak in cold water for a while.

Meanwhile, combine canola oil, ginger, vinegar, chili, salt, and pepper in a mixing bowl.

Drain well the asparagus and place in a large bowl and add spring onions and red cabbage. Drizzle with dressing and toss all well to coat. Serve immediately.

Nutrition information per serving: Kcal: 91, Protein: 4.3g, Carbs: 10.2g, Fats: 5.0g

16.   Choco Green Smoothie

Ingredients:

1 cup of coconut milk

½ cup of frozen blackberries

1 cup of fresh spinach, chopped

¼ cup of cocoa, raw

2 tbsp of honey

Preparation:

Combine all ingredients in a food processor and blend until nicely smooth. Transfer the mixture to a serving glasses and add a few ice cubes, or refrigerate for 30 minutes before serving.

Nutrition information per serving: Kcal: 383, Protein: 5.7g, Carbs: 33.8g, Fats: 30.3g

17. Barbunya Pilaki

Ingredients:

2 cups of cranberry beans (I used fresh, but you can use dried beans instead)

2 medium-sized onions, peeled and finely chopped

3 large carrots, cleaned and chopped

3 large tomatoes, peeled and finely chopped

3 tbsp of extra-virgin olive oil

A handful of fresh parsley

2 cups of water

Preparation:

Soak the beans overnight. Rinse and set aside.

Preheat 1 tablespoon of oil in a large saucepan over a medium-high temperature. add onions, and stir-fry for 5 minutes, or until translucent. Now, add the remaining oil and all other ingredients. Bring it to a boil, then reduce the heat to low. Cover with a lid and add more water to adjust thickness while cooking, if needed.

Cook for about 2 hours, or until set. Serve warm.

Nutrition information per serving: Kcal: 329, Protein: 16.5g, Carbs: 50.9g, Fats: 8.7g

18.   Mackerel with Greens

Ingredients:

4 medium-sized mackerels, skin on

1 lb of fresh spinach, torn

5 large potatoes, peeled and sliced

4 tbsp of olive oil

3 garlic cloves, crushed

1 tsp of dried rosemary, finely chopped

2 springs of fresh mint leaves, chopped

1 lemon, juiced

1 tsp of sea salt

Preparation:

Place the potatoes in a pot of boiling water. Sprinkle with some salt and cook for 5 minutes. Remove from the heat and drain. Set aside.

Preheat 2 tablespoons of oil in a deep pot over a medium-high temperature. Add spinach and cook for 2 minutes. now, place the potatoes in one layer, and top with fish. Pour the remaining oil and sprinkle with some salt, mint rosemary, salt, and garlic. Pour 1 cup of water, or more if needed to cover all ingredients. Cover with a lid and cook for 1 hour on low temperature.

Nutrition information per serving: Kcal: 244, Protein: 14g, Carbs: 19.2g, Fats: 12.4g

19.   Chicken Tighs with Potatoes

Ingredients:

4 chicken thighs, boneless

3 large potatoes, wedged

1 tbsp of freshly squeezed lemon juice

2 garlic cloves, crushed

1 tsp of ginger, ground

1 tbsp of cayenne pepper

1 tsp of fresh mint, finely chopped

¼ cup of olive oil

½ tsp of salt

Preparation:

In a small bowl, combine olive oil with lemon juice, crushed garlic, ground ginger, mint, cayenne pepper, and salt. Brush each chicken piece with this mixture and transfer to a heavy-bottomed pot.

Add potatoes, the remaining marinade, and 1 ½ cup of water.

Cover with a lid and set the heat to low. Cook for about 1-2 hours, or until the potatoes are fork-tender.

Remove from the pot to a serving plates and serve warm with some spring onions. This is, however, optional.

Nutrition information per serving: Kcal: 524, Protein: 37.8g, Carbs: 45.2g, Fats: 21.6g

20.   Sour Zucchini Stew

Ingredients:

4 medium-sized zucchini, peeled and sliced

1 large eggplant, peeled and chopped

3 medium-sized red bell peppers

½ cup fresh tomato juice

2 tsp of Italian seasoning

½ tsp of salt

2 tbsp of olive oil

Preparation:

Grease the bottom of a deep pot with olive oil. Now, add sliced zucchini and eggplant, red bell peppers, and tomato juice. Stir well and season with Italian seasoning, and salt. Give it a final stir and pour about ½ cup of water.

Cover with a lid and cook for about 1 hour over a low temperature. You want the zucchini to be fork tender, but not overcooked.

Remove from the heat and set aside to cool for a while. Serve as a cold salad, side dish, or keep in the refrigerator

Nutrition information per serving: Kcal: 132, Protein: 3.7g, Carbs: 18.1g, Fats: 6.8g

21.   Citrus Quinoa Porridge

Ingredients:

1 cup of white quinoa

2 tbsp of lemon juice, freshly squeezed

¼ tsp of salt

1 tsp of lemon zest, freshly grated

2 cups of vegetable stock, unsalted

1 tbsp of coconut oil

Preparation:

Combine quinoa and water in a medium pot. Bring it to a boil and then reduce the heat to low. Add lemon juice and butter. Sprinkle with lemon zest and a pinch of salt. Cover with a lid and cook for another 15 minutes. Remove from the heat and serve.

Nutrition information per serving: Kcal: 132, Protein: 3.7g, Carbs: 18.1g, Fats: 6.8g

22.   Eggplant Cheese Moussaka

Ingredients:

1 large eggplant, sliced

5 oz of Mozzarella cheese

3 ½ oz of kaymak cheese

2 medium-sized tomatoes, sliced

¼ cup of extra-virgin olive oil

1 tsp of salt

½ tsp of black pepper, freshly ground

1 tsp of oregano, dried

Preparation:

Grease the bottom of heavy-bottomed pot with 2 tablespoons of olive oil. Slice the eggplant and make a layer in the pot. Now, add one slice of mozzarella and then one slice of tomato on each eggplant. Top with eggplant and kaymak. You can repeat the process until you have used all the ingredients.

Meanwhile combine the remaining olive oil with salt, pepper, and dried oregano. Pour the mixture over the moussaka, add about ½ cup of water.

Cover with a lid and cook for about 1 hour. You don't want to overcook it because it will lose its shape. Serve immediately or even refrigerate overnight.

Nutrition information per serving: Kcal: 250, Protein: 11.7g, Carbs: 10.8g, Fats: 19.2g

23.   Marinated Tuna Steak

Ingredients:

¼ cup of fresh parsley, finely chopped

3 garlic cloves, minced

3 tbsp of lemon juice, freshly squeezed

½ cup of olive oil

4 tuna steaks

½ tsp of smoked paprika

½ tsp of cumin, ground

½ tsp of chili pepper, ground

½ tsp of Himalayan salt

¼ tsp of black pepper, ground

Preparation:

Place parsley, garlic, paprika, cumin, chili, salt, pepper and lemon juice in a food processor and pulse to combine. Gradually add in the oil and mix the ingredients until a smooth mixture.

Transfer the mixture into a bowl, add the fish and gently toss to coat the fish evenly with sauce. Chill for at least 2 hours to allow the flavors to penetrate into the fish.

Remove the fish from the chiller and preheat the grill. Lightly brush the grid with oil, place the fish and grill for about 3 to 4 minutes on each side.

Remove the fish from the grill, transfer on a serving plate and serve with lemon wedges or some vegetables

Nutrition information per serving: Kcal: 410, Protein: 30.4g, Carbs: 1.6g, Fats: 31.7g

24. Green Pineapple Smoothie

Ingredients:

¼ cup of fresh pineapple, chopped

1 cup of cucumber, peeled and chopped

1 kiwi, peeled and chopped

1 tsp of ginger, ground

1 cup of Iceberg lettuce

1 tbsp of honey, raw

2 cups of water

Preparation:

Combine all ingredients in a food processor and blend until nicely smooth.Transfer the mixture to a serving glasses and refrigerate for 1 hour before serving. Enjoy!

Nutrition information per serving: Kcal: 40, Protein: 0.6g, Carbs: 10.1g, Fats: 0.2g

25.   Meat Pie with Yogurt

Ingredients:

2 lb lean ground beef

5-6 garlic cloves, crushed

1 tsp of salt

½ tsp of black pepper, freshly ground

1 (16 oz) pack of yufka dough

½ cup of butter, melted

1 cup of sour cream

3 cups of liquid yogurt

Preparation:

Preheat the oven to 375°F.

In a large bowl, combine ground beef with garlic cloves, salt, and pepper. Mix well until fully incorporated.

Lay a sheet of yufka on a work surface and brush with melted butter. Line with the meat mixture and roll up. Repeat the process until you have used all the ingredients.

Gently place the pie pieces in a lightly greased baking sheet. Brushthe remaining butter over the prepared pie pieces.

Place it in the oven and bake for about 25-30 minutes. Remove from the oven and let it cool for a while.

Meanwhile, combine sour cream with yogurt. Spread the mixture over pie and serve cold.

Nutrition information per serving: Kcal: 503, Protein: 47.4g, Carbs: 2.6g, Fats: 32.8g

26. Cold Cauliflower Salad

Ingredients:

1 lb of cauliflower florets

1 lb of broccoli

4 garlic cloves, crushed

¼ cup of extra-virgin olive oil

1 tsp of salt

1 tbsp of dry rosemary, crushed

Preparation:

Rinse and drain the vegetables. Cut into bite-sized pieces and place in a deep pot. Add olive oil and 1 cup of water. Season with salt, crushed garlic and dry rosemary.

Cover with a lid and cook for 1 hour. Remove from the heat and transfer to a serving bowl. Chill well before serving.

Nutrition information per serving: Kcal: 182, Protein: 5.7g, Carbs: 15.1g, Fats: 13.2g

27. Garlic Meatballs

Ingredients:

1lb of lean ground beef

7oz of white rice

2 small onions, finely chopped

2 garlic cloves, crushed

1 egg, beaten

1 large potato, peeled and sliced

3 tbsp of extra-virgin olive oil

1 tsp of salt

Preparation:

In a large bowl, combine lean ground beef with rice, finely chopped onions, crushed garlic, one beaten egg, and salt. Shape the mixture into 15-20 meatballs, depending on the size.

Grease the bottom of a deep pot with olive oil. Make the first layer with slice potatoes and top with meatballs. Add water enough to cover all ingredients and bring it to a boil. Now, reduce the heat to low and cover with a lid.

Cook for 1 hour and then remove from the heat. Set aside to cool and serve with greek yogurt or steamed vegetables. However, this is optional.

Nutrition information per serving: Kcal: 468, Protein: 33.5g, Carbs: 47.4g, Fats: 15.3g

28. Moroccan Chickpea Soup

Ingredients:

14 oz chickpeas, soaked

2 large carrots, finely chopped

2 small onions, finely chopped

2 large tomatoes, peeled and finely chopped

3 tbsp of tomato paste

A handful of fresh parsley, finely chopped

2 cups of vegetable broth

3 tbsp of extra-virgin olive oil

1 tsp of salt

Preparation:

Soak the chickpeas overnight. Rinse and drain. Set side.

Grease the bottom of a deep pot with olive oil. Place the rinsed chickpeas, chopped onions, carrot, and finely chopped tomatoes.

Pour the vegetable broth and season with salt. Stir in tomato paste and add 1 cup of water. Bring it to a boil and add more water to adjust the thickness, if needed. Cover with a lid and cook for 2 hours on low temperature.

Sprinkle with fresh parsley and serve.

Nutrition information per serving: Kcal: 420, Protein: 18.9g, Carbs: 58.6g, Fats: 14.3g

29.   Mango Avocado Salad

Ingredients:

1 cup of avocado, peeled and chopped

1 cup of mango, chopped

½ cup of baby spinach, roughly chopped

1 tbsp of olive oil

2 tbsp of lemon juice, freshly squeezed

¼ tsp of chili pepper, ground

½ tsp of sea salt

¼ tsp of black pepper, ground

Preparation:

Combine spinach, oil, and spinach in a bowl. Toss to coat and set aside.

In a separate bowl, combine mango, avocado, chili, pepper, and salt. Now stir in this mixture into the bowl with spinach. Let it stand for 30 minutes before serving to allow flavors to mingle.

Nutrition information per serving: Kcal: 316, Protein: 3.2g, Carbs: 32.1g, Fats: 22.1g

30.   Wild Salmon with Spinach

Ingredients:

1 lb of wild salmon fillets, boneless

1 lb of fresh spinach, torn

4 tbsp of olive oil

2 garlic cloves, finely chopped

2 tbsp of lemon juice

1 tbsp of fresh rosemary, chopped

1 tsp of sea salt

¼ tsp of black pepper, ground

Preparation:

Preheat the olive oil in a large frying pan over a medium-high temperature. place the salmon fillets and sprinkle with rosemary, salt, and black pepper. Cook for 5 minutes on each side and remove from the heat. Sprinkle with lemon juice and set aside.

Meanwhile, place the spinach in a large pot. Add enough water to cover and bring it to a boil. Briefly, cook for about 2 minutes, or until greens are tender. Drain in a colander. Transfer the spinach to a serving plates. Top with salmon fillets and sprinkle with some more olive oil before serving, but this is optional.

Nutrition information per serving: Kcal: 432, Protein: 44.9g, Carbs: 2.1g, Fats: 28.3g

31.   Almond Spinach Smoothie

Ingredients:

1 cup of fresh spinach, finely chopped

¼ cup of frozen raspberries

¼ cup of almonds, roughly chopped

1 cup of almond milk

1 large banana, chopped

1 tbsp of honey, raw

Preparation:

Combine all ingredients in a food processor and blend until nicely smooth. Transfer to a serving glasses and refrigerate for 1 hour before serving.

Nutrition information per serving: Kcal: 315, Protein: 4.5g, Carbs: 28.1g, Fats: 23.2 g

32.   Stuffed Peppers

Ingredients:

2 lbs of green peppers

1 large onion, finely chopped

1 lb of lean ground beef

¼ cup of white rice

½ cup of fire-roasted tomatoes

1 medium-sized tomato, sliced

½ tsp of salt

1 tsp of Cayenne pepper, ground

3 tbsp of olive oil

¼ tsp of black pepper.

Preparation:

Cut the stem end of each pepper and remove the seeds. Rinse and set aside.

In a medium-sized bowl, combine meat with finely chopped onion, rice, tomatoes, salt, and cayenne pepper. Stir well to combine.

Use about 1-2 tablespoons of this mixture and fill each pepper, but make sure to leave at least ½ inch of headspace.

Grease the bottom of a heavy-bottomed deep pot with some oil. Make the first layer with tomato slices. Gently arrange the peppers and add two cups of water. Optionally, toss in a handful of green beans. Bring it to a boil, then reduce the heat to low and cover with a lid. Cook for about 1 hour on low temperature. Sprinkle with some pepper before serving.

Nutrition information per serving: Kcal: 410, Protein: 37.9g, Carbs: 24.7g, Fats: 18.2g

33.   Butter Veal Kebab

Ingredients:

2 lb veal shoulder, boneless, cut into bite-sized pieces

3 large tomatoes, roughly chopped

2 tbsp of all-purpose flour

3 tbsp of butter

1 tbsp of Cayenne pepper, ground

1 tsp of salt

1 tbsp of parsley, finely chopped

1 cup of Greek yogurt (can be replaced with sour cream), for serving

1 pide bread (can be replaced with any bread you have on hand)

Preparation:

Melt 2 tablespoons of butter in a deep pot over a medium-high temperature. Make a layer with veal chops and pour enough water to cover. Season with salt and bring it to a boil. Now, reduce the heat to low and simmer for 2 hours, or until meat fork-tender.

Melt the remaining butter in a small skillet. Add cayenne pepper, all-purpose flour, and briefly stir-fry - for about two minutes. Remove from the heat.

Chop pide bread and arrange on a serving plate. Place the meat and tomato on top. Drizzle with browned cayenne pepper, top with Greek yogurt and sprinkle with chopped parsley.

Serve immediately.

Nutrition information per serving: Kcal: 437, Protein: 49.7g, Carbs: 8.9g, Fats: 21.8g

34.   Fish Stew

Ingredients:

2 lbs of different fish and seafood

¼ cup of extra-virgin olive oil

2 large onions, finely chopped

2 large carrots, grated

A handful of fresh parsley, finely chopped

3 garlic cloves, crushed

3 cups of water (optionally 1 ½ cup of water and 1 ½ cup of dry white wine)

1 tsp of sea salt

Preparation:

Spread about 3 tablespoons of olive oil over the bottom of a heavy-bottomed pot. Add finely chopped onion and crushed garlic. Stir-fry for about 3-4 minutes, or until translucent. Now, add carrots and parsley. Stir well and cook for another 3-4 minutes.

Add the fish, water, and the remaining oil. Sprinkle with some salt and pepper to taste and bring it to a boil.

Reduce the temperature to low and cover with a lid. Cook for 1 hour, or until fish flake and easily break with a fork.

Sprinkle with a few drops of freshly squeezed lemon juice before serving, but this is optional.

Nutrition information per serving: Kcal: 504, Protein: 37.2g, Carbs: 8.1g, Fats: 35.5g

35.   Spinach Pie

Ingredients:

1 lb spinach, rinsed and finely chopped

½ cup of Mascarpone cheese

½ cup of Feta cheese, shredded

3 eggs, beaten

½ cup of goat's cheese

3 tbsp of butter

½ cup of milk

½ tsp of salt

1 pack (6 sheets) yufka dough

Oil for greasing

Preparation:

Preheat the oven to 400°F.

In a large bowl, combine spinach with eggs, mascarpone, feta, and goat's cheese. Add some salt, but be careful because cheese is already salted. Set aside.

Dust a clean surface with flour and unfold the sheet of yufka onto it. Using a rolling pin, roll the dough to fit your baking dish. Repeat the process with the remaining five sheets.

Combine milk and butter in a small skillet. Bring it to a boil and allow the butter to melt completely. If needed, add some more salt. Remove from the heat.

Grease your baking dish with oil. Place two yufka sheets and brush with milk mixture. Make the first layer of spinach mixture and cover with another two yufka sheets. Again, brush with some butter and milk mixture and repeat the process until you have used all the ingredients.

Butter and milk will gently soften your yufka dough which is highly recommendable to have a delicious pie.

Place it in the oven and bake for 25-30 minutes, or until golden brown and crisp. Serve warm with yogurt or sour cream. However, this is optional.

Nutrition information per serving: Kcal: 297, Protein: 16.6g, Carbs: 6.6g, Fats: 23.6g

36. Pepper Meat

Ingredients:

2 lbs of beef fillet or another tender cut

5 medium-sized onions, finely chopped

3 tbsp of tomato paste

2 tbsp of oil

1 tbsp of butter, melted

2 tbsp of fresh parsley, finely chopped

½ tsp of black pepper, freshly ground

1 tsp of salt

Preparation:

Preheat the oil in a large saucepan over a medium-high temperature. Add the onions and stir-fry for 2 minutes. Now, add meat and cook for 5 minutes more, stirring occasionally.

Add all other ingredients and pour about 2 cups of water. Bring it to a boil, then reduce the heat to low. Cover with a lid and cook for about 25-30 minutes, or until fork-tender.

When done, stir in melted butter and serve warm.

Nutrition information per serving: Kcal: 382, Protein: 47.3g, Carbs: 10.3g, Fats: 16.4g

37.   Braised Greens

Ingredients:

1 lb of Swiss chard, torn (keep the stems)

2 medium-sized potatoes, peeled and finely chopped

¼ cup of extra-virgin olive oil

1 tsp of salt

Preparation:

Place potatoes in a large, heavy-bottomed pot. Add enough water to cover and bring it to a boil. Briefly cook, for about 5 minutes. Now, add Swiss chard, olive oil, and sprinkle with some salt. Add one more cup of water and then reduce the heat to low. Cover with a lid and cook for 40 minutes, or until soften.

Serve with fish, meat, or as a main dish.

Nutrition information per serving: Kcal: 204, Protein: 3.8g, Carbs: 21.1g, Fats: 13.4g

38.   Apple Pie

Ingredients:

2 lbs of Zestar apples

¼ cup of honey

¼ cup of breadcrumbs

2 tsp of cinnamon, ground

3 tbsp of lemon juice, freshly squeezed

1 tsp of vanilla sugar

¼ cup of oil

1 egg, beaten

¼ cup of all-purpose flour

2 tbsp of flaxseeds

Pie dough

Preparation:

Preheat the oven to 375°F.

First, peel the apples and cut into bite- sized pieces. Transfer to a large bowl. I like to add lemon juice. It gives a nice sour flavor and it prevents the apples to change the color before cooking.

Now, add breadcrumbs, vanilla sugar, honey, and cinnamon. You can also add 1 teaspoon of ground nutmeg in the mixture. I personally avoid it because I like the classic cinnamon taste. But you can experiment a bit. Mix well the ingredients and set aside.

On a lightly floured surface roll out the pie dough making 2 circle-shaped crusts. Grease a baking sheet with some oil (or even melted butter) and place one pie crust in it. Spoon the apple mixture and cover with the remaining crust. Seal by crimping edges and brush with beaten egg.

I like to sprinkle the pie with flaxseeds. It adds some great nutritional values to it, but it also gives a bit of crunchy flavor I absolutely adore. This, however, is optional. Bake for 20 minutes, then reduce the temperature to 350°F. Bake for another 45 minutes, or until golden brown and crispy.

Nutrition information per serving: Kcal: 214, Protein: 2.8g, Carbs: 27.4g, Fats: 11.2g

39.   Banana Vanilla Frappuccino

Ingredients:

1 cup of almond milk

1 large banana, chopped

½ tsp of vanilla extract

1 tsp of cocoa, raw

1 tbsp of honey, raw

Preparation:

Combine all ingredients in a food processor and blend until nicely smooth. Add water to adjust thickness, if needed. Transfer to a serving glasses and refrigerate. Top with whipping cream, chocolate chips, or cocoa before serving. However, this is optional.

Nutrition information per serving: Kcal: 373, Protein: 3.7g, Carbs: 31.4g, Fats: 28.9g

40.   Roast Lamb

Ingredients:

2 lb of lamb leg

3 tbsp extra-virgin olive oil

2 tsp salt

Preparation:

Grease the bottom of a large nonstick saucepan with olive oil.

Rinse and generously season the meat with salt and place in the saucepan. Cover with a lid and cook for about 20-25 minutes on low temperature, or until the meat is tender and separates from the bones. Serve with fresh onions, or whatever you like. However, this is optional.

Nutrition information per serving: Kcal: 437, Protein: 49.7g, Carbs: 8.9g, Fats: 21.8g

41.   Aparagus Omelet

Ingredients:

6 large eggs, beaten

1 cup of asparagus,trimmed and chopped

2 tsp of olive oil

2 garlic cloves, minced

2 tbsp of skim milk

1 tbsp of chives, minced

1 tbsp of fresh parsley, finely chopped

1 tbsp of lemon juice, freshly squeezed

1 tsp of salt

¼ tsp of black pepper, ground

Preparation:

Combine eggs, milk, parsley, chives, salt and pepper in a mixing bowl. Whisk well with a for or hand mixer. Set aside.

Preheat the oil in a large frying pan over a medium-high temperature. Add garlic and stir-fry for 2 minutes. Add asparagus and about ½ cup of water. Cook until soften, or the liquid almost evaporates. Pour the egg mixture and spread evenly. Cook for about 2-3 minutes on each side. Remove from the heat and fold the omelet. Serve immediately.

Nutrition information per serving: Kcal: 188, Protein: 14.1g, Carbs: 4.0g, Fats: 13.2g

42.   Rosemary Meatballs with Yogurt

Ingredients:

1 lb lean ground beef

3 garlic cloves, crushed

¼ cup of all-purpose flour

1 tbsp of fresh rosemary, crushed

1 large egg, beaten

½ tsp of salt

3 tbsp of extra virgin olive oil

For serving:

2 cups of liquid yogurt

1 cup of Greek yogurt

2 tbsp of fresh parsley

1 garlic clove, crushed

Preparation:

In a large bowl, combine ground beef with crushed garlic, rosemary, one egg, and salt. Using a spoon or your hands, mix well to combine. I like to add some corn flour for extra crispiness, but this is totally optional.

Lightly dampen hands and shape 1 ½ inch balls transferring into a heavy-bottomed pot, as you work. Slowly add about ½ cup of water.

Bring it to a boil, then reduce the heat to low. Cover with a lid and cook for 10 minutes, or until nicely browned. Remove from the heat and set aside to cool completely.

Meanwhile, combine liquid yogurt with Greek yogurt, parsley, and crushed garlic. Stir well and drizzle over meatballs. Enjoy!

Nutrition information per serving: Kcal: 477, Protein: 49.6g, Carbs: 17.8g, Fats: 21.4g

43.   The Sultan's Soup

Ingredients:

3 ½ oz of carrots, finely chopped

3 ½ oz of celery root, finely chopped

A handful of green peas, soaked

A handful of fresh okra

2 tbsp of butter

2 tbsp of fresh parsley, finely chopped

1 egg yolk

2 tbsp of kaymak cheese

¼ cup of lemon juice, freshly squeezed

1 bay leaf

1 tsp of salt

½ tsp of black pepper, ground

4 cups of beef broth, plus one cup of water

Preparation:

Melt the butter in a large saucepan over a medium-high temperature. Add carrots, cellery, okra, parsley, and peas. Stir well and cook for 5 minutes, or until slightly soften.

Now, pour the beef broth and water. Stir well and sprinkle salt and pepper. Bring it to a boil and then reduce the heat to low. Add bay leaf, egg jolk, and lemon juice. Cook for about 1 hour, or until vegetables tender. Stir in the cheese and cook for 2 more minutes.

Remove from the heat and serve immediately.

Nutrition information per serving: Kcal: 161, Protein: 2.8g, Carbs: 9.1g, Fats: 13.4g

44.   Potato Moussaka

Ingredients:

2 lb large potatoes, peeled and sliced

1 lb lean ground beef

1 large onion, peeled and finely chopped

1 tsp of salt

½ tsp of black pepper, ground

½ cup of milk

2 large eggs, beaten

Vegetable oil

Sour cream or Greek yogurt, for serving

Preparation:

Preheat the oven to 400°F.

Grease the bottom of a large baking dish with some vegetable oil. Make one layer with sliced potatoes and brush with some milk. Spread the ground beef and make another layer with potatoes. Brush well with the remaining milk and add ½ cup of water. Cover with aluminum foil and place it in the oven.

Bake for 40 minutes, or until potatoes are golden brown. Now, spread the beaten eggs evenly and return in the oven for 10 more minutes. When done, top with some sour cream or Greek yogurt and serve!

Nutrition information per serving: Kcal: 458, Protein: 34.9g, Carbs: 36.2g, Fats: 19.2g

45. Black Seafood Pasta

Ingredients:

1 lb of fresh seafood mix

¼ cup of extra-virgin olive oil

4 garlic cloves, crushed

1 tbsp of fresh parsley, finely chopped

1 tsp of fresh rosemary, finely chopped

½ cup of white wine

1 tsp of salt

1 lb squid ink pasta

Preparation:

Preheat the oil in a large saucepan over a medium-high temperature. Add garlic and stir-fry until translucent. Add seafood mix and sprinkle with rosemary, parsley, and salt. Stir all well and cook for 4-5 minutes.

Now, stir in the wine and pour about ½ cup of water. Bring it to a boil, then reduce the heat to low. Cover with a lid and cook for 15-20 minutes, or until set. Remove from the heat and set aside.

Use a package instructions to prepare pasta. Squid ink pasta usually doesn't take more than 5 minutes in a pot of boiling water, so be careful not to overcook it. Remove from the heat and stir in the seafood mix. Serve!

Nutrition information per serving: Kcal: 273, Protein: 26.1g, Carbs: 3.8g, Fats: 14.6g

46.   Cinnamon Flaxseed Smoothie

Ingredients:

1 cup of almond milk, unsweetened

1 tsp of vanilla extract

1 large apple, cored and chopped

1 tbsp of honey, raw

Preparation:

Combine all ingredients in a food processor and blend until nicely smooth. Transfer to a serving glasses and refrigerate 30 minutes before serving.

Nutrition information per serving: Kcal: 372, Protein: 3.1g, Carbs: 31.0g, Fats: 28.8g

47. Spicy White Peas

Ingredients:

1 lb of white peas

1 large onion, finely chopped

1 small chili pepper, finely chopped

2 tbsp of all-purpose flour

2 tbsp of butter

1 tbsp of Cayenne pepper, ground

3 bay leaves, dried

1 tsp of salt

½ tsp of black pepper, freshly ground

Preparation:

Melt the butter in a large skillet over a medium-high temperature. Add chopped onion and stir-fry for 5 minutes, or until translucent.

Now, add peas, finely chopped chili pepper, bay leaves, salt, and pepper. Gently stir in the flour and cayenne pepper. Pour about 3 cups of water.

Bring it to a boil and then reduce the heat to low. Cover with a lid and cook for 45 minutes. Remove from the heat and serve.

Nutrition information per serving: Kcal: 177, Protein: 7.2g, Carbs: 23.9g, Fats: 6.5g

48.   Stuffed Onions

Ingredients:

10-12medium-sized sweet onions, peeled

1 lb of lean ground beef

½ cup of rice

3 tbsp of olive oil

1 tbsp of dry mint, ground

1 tsp of Cayenne pepper, ground

½ tsp of cumin, ground

1 tsp of salt

½ cup of tomato paste

½ cup Italian-style bread crumbs

A handful of fresh parsley, finely chopped

Preparation:

Cut a¼-inch slice from top of each onion and trim a small amount from the bottom end, This will make the onions stand upright. Place onions in a microwave-safe dish and add about 1 cup of water. Cover with a tight lid and microwave on HIGH 10-12 minutes or until onions are tender. Remove onions from a dish and cool slightly. Now carefully remove inner layers of onions with paring knife, leaving about a ¼-inch onion shell.

In a large bowl, combine ground beef with rice, olive oil, mint, cayenne pepper, cumin, salt, and bread crumbs. Use 1 tablespoon of the mixture to fill the onions.

Grease the bottom of a deep pot with some oil and place stuffed onions. Add about 2 ½ cups of water and cover with a lid. Cook for about 45-50 minutes on low temperature. Remove from the heat.

Sprinkle with chopped parsley or even arugula and serve with sour cream and pide bread.

Nutrition information per serving: Kcal: 464, Protein: 34.3g, Carbs: 48.4g, Fats: 15.2g

49.   Warm Winter Compote

Ingredients:

1 lb of fresh figs

7 oz of Turkish figs

7 oz of fresh cherries, pitted

7 oz of plums, pitted

3 ½ oz of raisins

3 large apples, corred and chopped

3 tbsp of cornstarch

1 tsp of cinnamon, ground

1 tbsp of cloves

3 tbsp of honey

1 lemon, juiced

3 cups of water

Preparation:

Combine all ingredients in a deep pot. add about 3-4 cups of water (depending on how much liquid you wish). Bring it to a boil and then reduce the heat to low. Cook for 20 minutes, or until fruit is fork tender.

Nutrition information per serving: Kcal: 215, Protein: 2.2g, Carbs: 55.6g, Fats: 0.8g

50.   Mushroom Basil Omelet

Ingredients:

1 cup of button mushrooms, chopped

6 large eggs, beaten

2 garlic cloves, crushed

1 small onion, finely chopped

3 tbsp of skim milk

1 tbsp of extra-virgin olive oil

½ tsp of fresh rosemary, finely chopped

½ tsp of salt

¼ tsp of black pepper, ground

Preparation:

Combine eggs, milk, salt and pepper in a mixing bowl. Whisk with a fork to mix and set aside.

Preheat the oil in a large saucepan over a medium-high temperature. Add garlic and onion and stir-fry for 3 minutes. Now, add chopped mushrooms and cook until soften or heated trough. Pour the egg mixture and stir well. Cook for 5 minutes, or until eggs are set. Stir with a wooden spoon and scrap the bottom a of a saucepan and cook for 5 minutes, or until eggs are set.

Nutrition information per serving: Kcal: 207, Protein: 14.2g, Carbs: 5.4g, Fats: 14.7g

51.   Brussels Sprout Cream Soup

Ingredients:

1lb fresh brussel sprouts, halved

7oz fresh baby spinach, torn

1 tsp of sea salt

1 cup of whole milk

3 tbsp of sour cream

1 tbsp of fresh celery, finely chopped

2 cups of water

1 tbsp of butter

Preparation:

Melt the butter in a large skillet over a medium-high temperature. Add spinach and Brussels sprouts and about 2 tablespoons of water to prevent sticking to the pan. Sprinkle with some salt and cook for 3-4 minutes, or until slightly tender.

Now, add milk, sour cream, celery, and water. Bring it to a boil then reduce the heat to low and cook for about 15-20 minutes, covered. Remove from the heat and let it cool for a while. Transfer the mixture to a food processor and blend until smooth. Heat up the soup again and serve.

Nutrition information per serving: Kcal: 194, Protein: 10.2g, Carbs: 21.7g, Fats: 9.8g

52.   Beef Stew with Eggplants

Ingredients:

10 oz of beef neck, or another tender cut, chopped into bite-sized pieces

1 large eggplant, sliced

2 cups of fire-roasted tomatoes

½ cup of fresh green peas

1 cup of beef broth

4 tbsp of olive oil

2 tbsp of tomato paste

1 tbsp of Cayenne pepper, ground

½ tsp of chili pepper, ground (optional)

½ tsp of salt

Parmesan cheese

Preparation:

Grease the bottom of a deep pot with olive oil. Toss all ingredients in it and add about 1-1 ½ cup of water. Bring it to a boil and then reduce the heat to low. Cover with a lid and cook for about 2 hours, or until the meat is fork-tender.

Sprinkle with Parmesan cheese before serving, but this is optional.

Nutrition information per serving: Kcal: 195, Protein: 15.3g, Carbs: 9.6g, Fats: 11.1g

53.　Green Tea Avocado Smoothie

Ingredients:

1 cup of Greek yogurt

½ cup of avocado, peeled

1 tsp of green tea, (1 tea bag)

1 tbsp of honey, raw

2 tbsp of hot water

1 tbsp of mint

Preparation:

Combine tea with hot water in a small cup or a bowl. Soak for 2 minutes.

Meanwhile, combine all the remaining ingredients except mint and add tea mixture. Blend until nicely smooth and transfer to a serving glasses. Refrigerate for 1 hour and garnish with mint before serving.

Nutrition information per serving: Kcal: 176, Protein: 9.9g, Carbs: 15.7g, Fats: 9.0g

54.   Stuffed Collard Greens

Ingredients:

1 ½ lb of collard greens, steamed

1 lb of lean ground beef

2 small onions, finely chopped

½ cup long grain rice

2 tbsp of olive oil

1 tsp of salt

½ tsp of black pepper, freshly ground

1 tsp of mint leaves, finely chopped

Preparation:

Boil a large pot of water and gently the greens. Briefly cook, for 2-3 minutes. Drain and gently squeeze the greens and set aside.

In a large bowl, combine the ground beef with finely chopped onions, rice, salt, pepper, and mint leaves.

Grease the bottom of a heavy-bottomed pot with some oil. Place leaves on your work surface, vein side up. Use 1 tablespoon of the meat mixture and place it in the bottom center of each leaf. Fold the sides over and roll up tightly. Tuck in the sides and gently transfer to a pot.

Cover with a lid and cook for 1 hour. Add more water if needed, while cooking.

Remove from the heat and serve.

Nutrition information per serving: Kcal: 156, Protein: 5.2g, Carbs: 21.0g, Fats: 7.4g

55.   Lemon Tuna Salad

Ingredients:

1 can of tuna, minced

4 tbsp of lemon juice, freshly squeezed

¼ cup of cream cheese

1 tbsp of fresh basil, finely chopped

3 tbsp of extra-virgin olive oil

1 cup of Iceberg lettuce, roughly chopped

1 tsp of salt

¼ tsp of black pepper, ground

¼ tsp of red pepper flakes

Preparation:

Preheat the oil in a large nonstick frying pan over a medium-high temperature. Add tuna, lemon juice, and sprinkle with basil, salt, black pepper, and red pepper flakes. Stir well and cook for 2 minutes.

Meanwhile, place lettuce and basil in a large bowl. Remove the tuna from the heat and transfer the mixture to a bowl directly from the pan with all juices. Stir in the cream cheese and serve immediately.

Nutrition information per serving: Kcal: 460, Protein: 26.3g, Carbs: 2.6g, Fats: 38.6g

56.   Whole Chicken & Veggies Stew

Ingredients:

1 whole chicken, (about 3 lbs)

10 oz of fresh broccoli

7 oz cauliflower florets

1 large onion, finely chopped

1 large potato, peeled and chopped

3 medium-sized carrots, sliced

1 large tomato, peeled and chopped

A handful of yellow wax beans, whole

A handful of fresh parsley, finely chopped

¼ cup of extra virgin olive oil

2 tsp of salt

½ tsp of black pepper, freshly ground

1 tbsp of Cayenne pepper, ground

Preparation:

Preheat the oven to 450°F.

Clean the chicken and generously sprinkle with some salt. Set aside.

Preheat the oil in a large skillet over a medium-high temperature. Add onion and stir-fry for 3-4 minutes, or until translucent. Add carrot and continue to cook for another 5 minutes.

Now, add broccoli, cauliflower, potato, tomato, beans and parsley. Stir all well and cook for 2-3 minutes. Transfer all to a large baking dish and top with chicken. Sprinkle with some Cayenne pepper, black pepper and place it in the oven.

Bake for about 10-15 minutes, then reduce the heat to 350°F. Bake for about 45-50 minutes, or until set.

Nutrition information per serving: Kcal: 290, Protein: 31.2g, Carbs: 39.4g, Fats: 6.5g

57.   Mediterranean Grilled Trout

Ingredients:

4oz fresh trout, cleaned

¼ cup of parsley, finely chopped

2 garlic cloves, crushed

¼ cup of lemon juice, freshly squeezed

½ teaspoon smoked paprika

1 tbsp of fresh rosemary, finely chopped

½ teaspoon chili pepper, ground

½ tsp of black pepper, freshly ground

¼ cup of olive oil

Preparation:

Mix together parsley, garlic, paprika, chili, lemon juice, and olive oil in a large bowl. Place the fish in this marinade and coat well. Set aside for 1 hour to allow flavors to penetrate into the fish.

Remove the fish from the refrigerator and preheat the grill pan. Place the fish and grill for about 3 to 4 minutes on each side.

Remove the fish from the grill, transfer on a serving plate and serve with lemon or some vegetables of your choice.

Nutrition information per serving: Kcal: 143, Protein: 21.5g, Carbs: 0.6g, Fats: 7.7g

58.   Salmon Cilantro Pesto

Ingredients

1 lbs of salmon fillets, cut into bite-sized pieces

1 cup of fresh cilantro, finely chopped

5 tbsp of olive oil

2 garlic cloves, minced

4 tbsp of Parmesan cheese, grated

3 tbsp of almonds, roughly chopped

½ tsp of sea salt

Preparation:

Preheat 1 tablespoon of oil in a large saucepan over a medium-high temperature. Add 1 minced garlic clove and stir-fry for 2 minutes. Now, add meat and cook for about 5-7minutes, or until its doneness. Set aside.

Meanwhile, combine remaining garlic, cilantro, cheese, almonds, and sea salt in a food processor. Blend for 1 minute, then gradually add oil and blend until incorporated.

Spoon the pesto over the salmon, or serve as a dip for salmon chops.

Nutrition information per serving: Kcal: 465, Protein: 33.5g, Carbs: 2.4g, Fats: 37.4g

59.   Stuffed Portobello

Ingredients:

6 large portobello mushrooms,

½ cup of fresh basil, finely chopped

1 cup of fresh arugula, chopped

4 tbsp of fresh parsley, finely chopped

4 tbsp of Parmesan cheese

2 garlic cloves, minced

2 oz of tomatoes, sun-dried

¼ cup of olive oil

¼ tsp of black pepper, ground

½ tsp of sea salt

Preparation:

Preheat the oven to 400°F.

Clean the mushroom stems and scrap the gills as much as you can to make a small caps.

Preheat the grill over a medium temperature. Place the mushrooms and grill for 3 minutes on each side. Remove from the grill and set aside.

Meanwhile, combine arugula, basil, cheese, tomatoes, garlic, oil, pepper, and salt in a food processor. Pulse until well combined.

Now, spoon this mixture into a mushroom caps. Place some baking paper over a large baking dish and spread the stuffed mushrooms. Place it in the oven for 2-3 minutes, or until cheese melts. Remove from the oven and serve immediately.

Nutrition information per serving: Kcal: 192, Protein: 4.9g, Carbs: 4.0g, Fats: 18.9g

60. Blueberry Kale Smoothie

Ingredients:

½ cup of frozen blueberries

½ cup of fresh kale, roughly chopped

½ cup of red cabbage, chopped

1 cup of water

Preparation:

Combine all ingredients in a food processor and pulse until nicely smooth. Transfer the mixture to a serving glasses and add a few ice cubes or refrigerate before serving.

Nutrition information per serving: Kcal: 33, Protein: 1.0g, Carbs: 8.0g, Fats: 0.1g

61.   Oven-Baked Cod

Ingredients:

1 lb of cod fish, cut into fillets, skinless and boneless

1 tsp of sea salt

½ tsp of black pepper, ground

3 tbsp of olive oil

1 tbsp of vinegar

1 cup of spinach, chopped into bite-sized pieces

Preparation:

Preheat the oven to 375°F.

Place the spinach in a pot of boiling water. Cook until fork-tender. Remove from the heat and drain well. Set aside to cool.

Combine vinegar, salt, pepper, and 2 tablespoons of olive oil in a mixing bowl.

Place some baking paper in a large baking sheet. Grease with the remaining olive oil and place the fish. Sprinkle with some salt and place it in the oven. Bake for about 10-12 minutes, then add spinach. Sprinkle all with dressing and bake for another 3-4 minutes. Remove from the oven and let it cool for a while.

Nutrition information per serving: Kcal: 283, Protein: 34.9g, Carbs: 0.6g, Fats: 15.3g

62.   Green Beans and Mushrooms

Ingredients:

1 lb of green beans, chopped

1 cup of button mushrooms, chopped

2 tbsp of fresh parsley, finely chopped

1 medium-sized onion, chopped

2 tbsp of olive oil

½ tsp of salt

¼ tsp of black pepper, ground

Preparation:

Place the beans in a pot of boiling water and cook for about 10 minutes, or until soften. Remove from the heat and drain. Set aside.

Preheat the oil in a large saucepan over a medium-high temperature. Add onion and stir-fry for 3 minutes. Now, add mushrooms and sprinkle with parsley, salt, and pepper. Add about 3-4 tablespoons of water to prevent sticking to the pan and cook for 5 minutes. Add beans and and stir all to combine. Cook for another 2-3 minutes.

Sprinkle with more salt or pepper, if needed. Remove from the heat and serve.

Nutrition information per serving: Kcal: 148, Protein: 4.0g, Carbs: 15.2g, Fats: 9.7g

63.   Apple Cinnamon Oatmeal

Ingredients:

1 cup of oatmeal

1 cup of almond milk

¼ cup of prunes, finely chopped

1 medium-sized apple, chopped

½ tsp of cinnamon, ground

1 tbsp of honey

Preparation:

Place oatmeal in a medium-sized bowl. Stir in the milk, prunes, cinnamon, and honey. Let it soak for about 10-15 minutes. Now, add chopped apple and stir all to combine and serve.

Nutrition information per serving: Kcal: 382, Protein: 6.0g, Carbs: 48.3g, Fats: 21.0g

64.   Lentil Lemon Salad

Ingredients:

1 cup of lentils, pre-cooked

3 cups of vegetable broth

2 cups of fresh arugula, chopped

½ cup of green onions, chopped

¼ cup of lemon juice, freshly squeezed

3 tbsp of fresh cilantro, finely chopped

1 tsp of fresh mint, finely chopped

½ tsp of Himalayan salt

¼ tsp of black pepper, ground

Preparation:

Combine lentils and vegetable stock in a deep pot. Bring it to a a boil and then reduce the heat to low. Cover with a lid and cook for about 50 minutes, or until lentils soften. Remove from the heat and drain well. Transfer to a large bowl.

Stir in the lemon juice, spring onions, cilantro, pepper, and himalayan salt. Throw a bunch of arugula on a serving plate and spoon the salad on top and serve.

Nutrition information per serving: Kcal: 139, Protein: 11.1g, Carbs: 20.9g, Fats: 1.2g

65.   Mushroom Spaghetti in Tomato Sauce

Ingredients:

8 oz of button mushrooms, chopped

10 oz of spaghetti

2 garlic cloves, crushed

1 lb of tomatoes, diced

½ tsp of chili pepper, ground

1 small onion, finely chopped

2 tbsp of vegetable oil

2 tbsp of fresh parsley, finely chopped

½ tsp of salt

¼ tsp of black pepper, ground

Preparation:

Prepare the spaghetti using package instructions. Drain well and set aside.

Preheat the oil in a large saucepan over a medium-high temperature. Add mushrooms and cook for about 3-4 minutes, or until slightly tender. Add garlic and parsley and continue to cook for another minute. Transfer all to a bowl and reserve the pan.

Throw in the onions and stir-fry until translucent. Add tomatoes and sprinkle with some chili and salt. Cook for about 10-12 minutes, or until thickened.

Stir in the tomato sauce into a bowl with spaghetti and top with mushrooms.

Nutrition information per serving: Kcal: 205, Protein: 7.4g, Carbs: 31.6g, Fats: 5.9g

66.   Chicken in Honey & Mustard

Ingredients:

1 lb of chicken breasts, thinly sliced

3 tbsp of honey, raw

3 tbsp of yellow mustard

1 tsp of dried basil, ground

½ tsp of sea salt

¼ tsp of red pepper, ground

Preparation:

Preheat the oven to 375°F.

In a bowl, combine meat, salt, and pepper. Rub with your hands to coat well.

Mix together mustard, honey, and basil. Add an extra pinch of salt to taste and stir well. Set aside.

Place aluminum foil on the bottom of a large baking dish. Spread the meat and spoon about half of the mustard mixture on top. Place it in the oven and bake for about 25-30 minutes. Now, turn over and spread the remaining half of the mixture. Bake it for 15 minutes, or until set.

Remove from the oven and set aside to cool for a while before serving.

Nutrition information per serving: Kcal: 365, Protein: 44.6g, Carbs: 18.9g, Fats: 11.8g

67.   Ginger Date Smoothie

Ingredients:

1 cup of skim milk

½ cup of dates, pitted

¼ tsp of ginger, ground

¼ tsp of nutmeg, ground

¼ tsp of cinnamon, ground

Preparation:

Combine all ingredients in a food processor and blend until nicely smooth. Transfer to a serving glases and refrigerate for at least 30 minutes before serving.

Nutrition information per serving: Kcal: 173, Protein: 5.1g, Carbs: 39.9g, Fats: 0.3g

68.   Turkey Broccoli Soup

Ingredients:

1 lb of turkey fillets, cut into bite-sized pieces

10 oz of broccoli, chopped

4 cups of vegetable stock

1 cup of skim milk

1 tbsp of butter

½ cup of cheddar cheese

¼ tsp of salt

¼ tsp of black pepper, ground

Preparation:

Place the broccoli in a pot of boiling water and cook until fork tender. Remove from the heat and drain well. Transfer to a food processor and add milk. Sprinkle with some salt and pepper and blend until creamy. Set aside.

Melt the butter in a large saucepan over a medium-high temperature. Add onion and stir-fry until translucent. Now, add turkey and cook for 5-7 minutes, until golden brown. Remove from the heat and set aside.

Pour vegetable stock in a deep pot and bring it to a boil. Add meat and broccoli mixture. Cook for 5 minutes and stir in the cheese. Remove from the heat and set aside to cool for a while before serving.

Nutrition information per serving: Kcal: 164, Protein: 20.6g, Carbs: 4.4g, Fats: 6.8g

69.   Watermelon Spinach Salad

Ingredients:

2 cups of watermelon, seeded

2 cups of fresh spinach, roughly chopped

½ cup of Feta cheese, crumbled

1 small red onion, chopped

4 tbsp of red wine vinegar

1 tbsp of extra-virgin olive oil

1 tbsp of fresh mint, minced

¼ tsp of Himalayan pink salt

¼ tsp of black pepper, ground

Preparation:

Mix together vinegar, olive oil, mint, salt, and pepper in a mixing bowl or a jar. Stir well, or close the lid and shake to mix. Set aside.

Combine watermelon, spinach, onion, and cheese in a large bowl. Drizzle with previously made marinade and toss to coat all well. Refrigerate for 1 hour before serving. Enjoy!

Nutrition information per serving: Kcal: 156, Protein: 5.1g, Carbs: 12.0g, Fats: 10.2g

70.   Parmesan Omelet

Ingredients:

4 large eggs

¼ cup of Parmesan cheese, crumbled

1 tbsp of fresh parsley, finely chopped

1 tbsp of fresh basil, finely chopped

2 tsp of butter

½ tsp of kosher salt

¼ tsp of black pepper, ground

Preparation:

Whisk all ingredients in a large bowl and set aside.

Melt the butter in a medium frying pan over a medium-high temperature. pour the egg mixture and cook for 4 minutes. Now, flip the omelet and cook for 2 more minutes. Remove from the heat and fold the omelet before serving.

Nutrition information per serving: Kcal: 448, Protein: 33.4g, Carbs: 3.1g, Fats: 34.6g

ADDITIONAL TITLES FROM THIS AUTHOR

70 Effective Meal Recipes to Prevent and Solve Being Overweight: Burn Fat Fast by Using Proper Dieting and Smart Nutrition

By

Joe Correa CSN

48 Acne Solving Meal Recipes: The Fast and Natural Path to Fixing Your Acne Problems in Less Than 10 Days!

By

Joe Correa CSN

41 Alzheimer's Preventing Meal Recipes: Reduce or Eliminate Your Alzheimer's Condition in 30 Days or Less!

By

Joe Correa CSN

70 Effective Breast Cancer Meal Recipes: Prevent and Fight Breast Cancer with Smart Nutrition and Powerful Foods

By

Joe Correa CSN